Winter Essential Oils

Winter and Spring Blends for Diffusers

Table of Contents

Introduction: Essential Oils for Diffusers?

With a title like this, you already know that this book is going to place a heavy emphasis on the importance of using essential oils for diffusers. But there are many methods of application when it comes to essential oils, so why do we stress the use of diffusers? Just think back to when you were a kid and your mom used to use special air fresheners and incense to make the house smell a little bit better?

I mean, forget about the febreze, we're talking about the heavy duty stuff; those powerful vanillas and scented candles that were only put out when company came over. Well guess what? That was aromatherapy my friends, and it was accomplishing much the same thing that diffusers accomplish, setting the backdrop for a strong scent to invade your senses and help you feel better!

In this book we are going to delve into some of the best essential oils for what ails you and the best methods of diffuser application in order to implement the healing properties of these great oils into your daily life. The sense of smell is a powerful ally in health, your nose works as a direct interface to your brain, and this is why essential oils work so great with diffusers.

Chapter 1: Winter Oils for Fatigue, Anxiety and Depression

Anxiety is a chronic problem in the modern world and unfortunately, in the stress filled world of today, many of us turn to self medication in order to treat our anxiety, often leading to alcoholism and drug addiction. Especially in the winter months. But you don't have to pop pills and drink alcohol in order to find that sense of calm you so desperately desire, because there are many essential oils that can help calm your nerves on a holistic level, calming your mind and body all in quick succession. Keep reading this chapter to find out more.

Angelica Oil

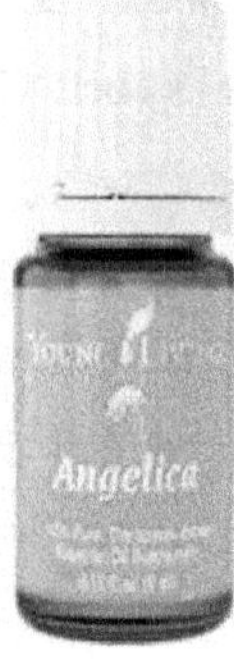

During the course of the winter months many of us feel stressed out. We feel it deep down in our muscles and even in our throbbing joints as we trudge through the ice and snow of another cold winter season. You could say that many factors are against you during the winter months. As the sun retreats earlier, and earlier in the day, there is a seasonal affective disorder (SAD) that makes many of us depressed and just a general overall exhaustion that makes us perpetually anxious.

Fortunately for us however, if we would just load up a few drops of angelica essential oil into our diffusers, we would start feeling a whole lot better. Along with relieving generalized anxiety, and helping those who breathe it relax, the aroma of angelica oil has also been known to help women reverse the effects of having an off course menstrual cycle.

This essential oil has a great aroma, reminiscent of a wooded forest, and provides a great backdrop during the winter months. I always enjoy this essential oil when it gets cold out. Put this essential oil in your diffuser and you will see much of your anxiety, depression and discomfort during the winter months completely disappear.

Geranium Oil

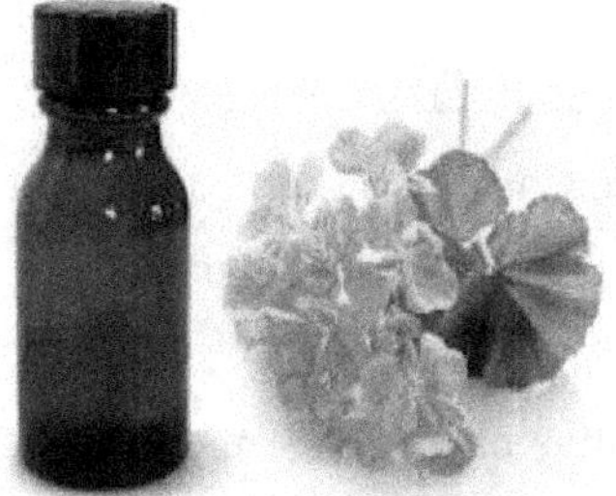

During the winter, many of us our more tired than anything else. The sun goes down much sooner and the nights are much longer, with this substantial lack of sunlight, we find ourselves in a state of constant fatigue. Geranium oil however has the ability of not only relieving your fatigue but it also puts you in a restive, good mood! This is especially important for those that suffer from Season Affective Disorder, because a good whiff of Geranium oil can chase those winter blues right away! Keep a hefty supply of this oil on stock for the whole duration of the winter!

Rose Oil

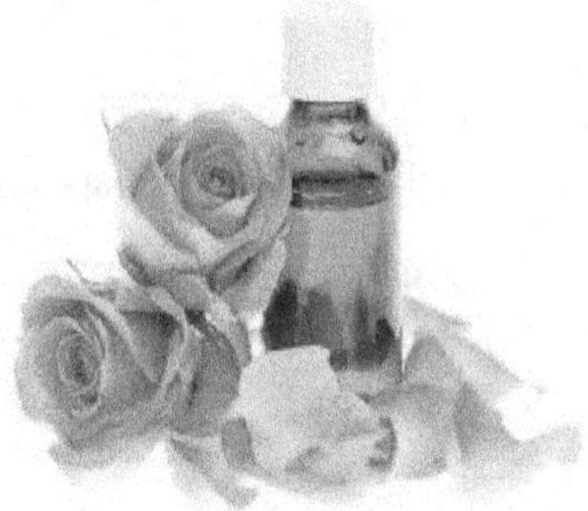

This oil is extracted directly from that flower that we all know and love; the rose. Violets are blue and roses are red, and this essential oil can really relieve that bad feeling in your head! Rose oil calms the mind, and relieves the restless, anxious fatigue that is so common during the winter months. It's also been known to cure headaches, which is a great added benefit for many winter migraine sufferers, providing a healthier alternative to over the counter headache medicine.

Studies have also shown that a regular routine of rose oil can even treat high blood pressure and rapid heart beats. This oil manages to calm the whole cardiovascular system. Priming it and putting it in a much better position to stave off any irregularities of the heart. For those that suffer from hypertension this is some particularly good news. So if you are feeling at odds this winter, just put a few drops of this essential oil in your diffuser, and you can fine tune your whole body!

Frankincense Oil

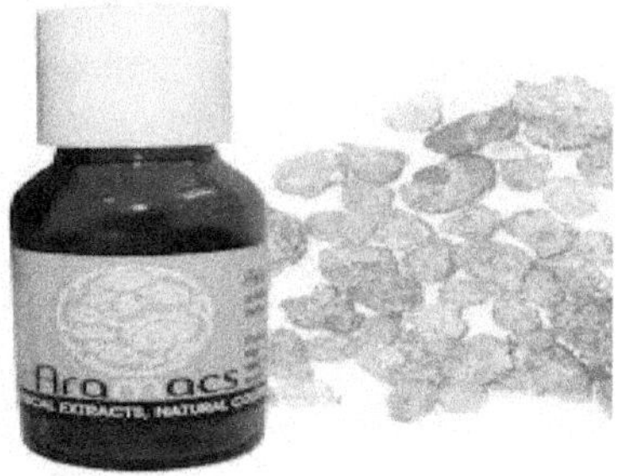

Just like the Christmas story of old told us, winter wouldn't be complete with some Frankincense and Myrrh. But it's frankincense in particular that has such a great knack for relieving depression and anxiety. Frankincense has been used for thousands of years in religious ceremonies, and this fact is no coincidence by any means.

Religious adherents prized burning frankincense as incense because of the relaxed meditative state that it would put them and their fellow parishioners in. You can benefit from this same relaxed state of mind too. Just put some of this wonderful oil in your diffuser and start your own aromatic routine with frankincense oil today. Your health will thank you for it!

Jasmine Oil

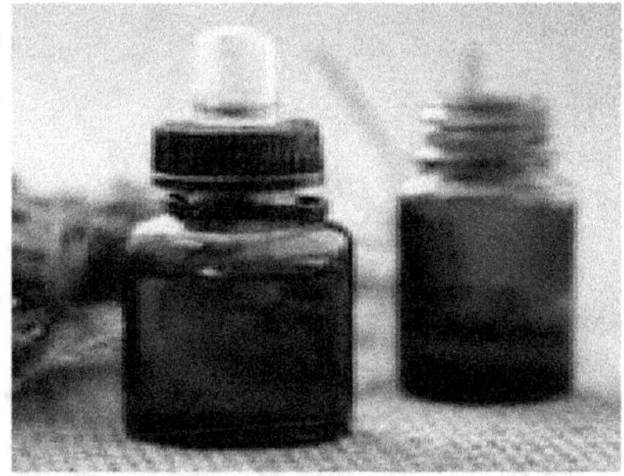

Winter can be exhausting, but this essential oil can give you just the right kind of boost to keep you going. The aroma of this oil eliminates fatigue and invigorates the whole body with energy. Jasmine oil is taken directly from Jasmine petals and condensed down into a highly concentrated form. Just a few drops in your diffuser should be enough to see a noticeable difference in your state of mind during the winter.

Neroli Oil

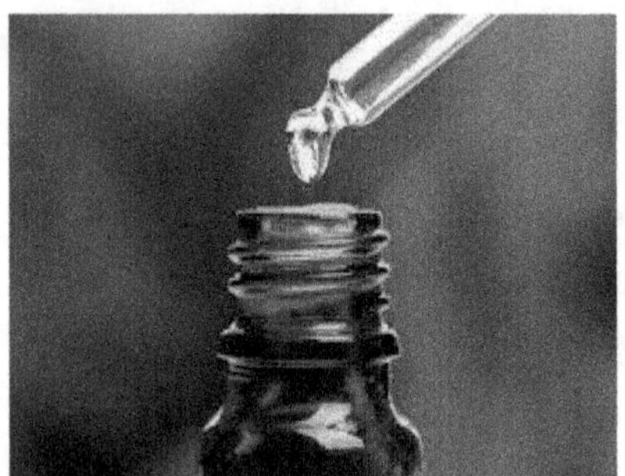

We all can get anxious during the winter, especially when it come to all the shopping, and hustle and bustle of the holiday season. Neroli can soothe those nerves, and even improve your mental focus. Brain fog dissipates as soon as you start burning neroli in your diffuser. If you need to have mental clarity this winter, put some of this oil in your diffuser as soon as you can.

Tangerine Oil

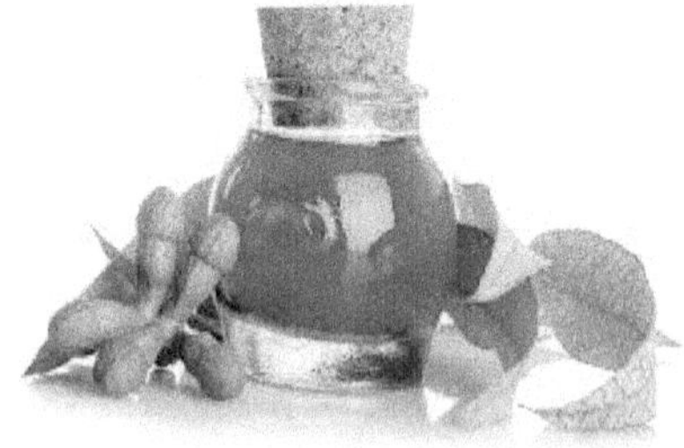

This oil derived, from the citrus fruit, is great at relieving anxiety and reducing fatigue. When breathed into the nose, it also works to clean out your respiratory system, as special anti-oxidizing agents work their way through your body. I myself have asthma, and I have witnessed the great affect that this essential oil has had on my own respiratory system. So be sure to give this essential oil a try in your diffuser.

Chamomile Oil

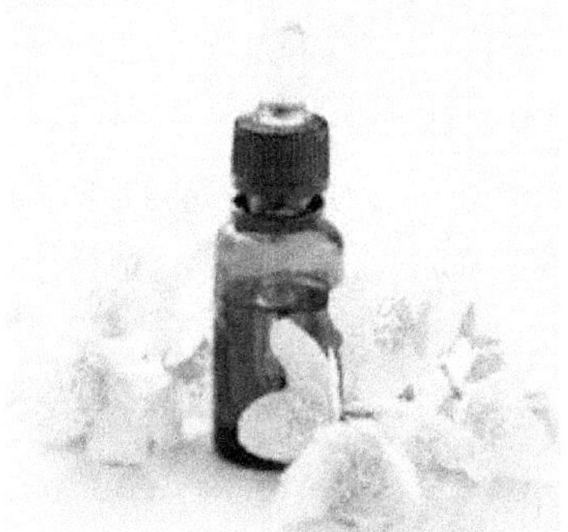

Chamomile is quite popular nowadays, you find it in tea, you find it in soaps, and shampoos, and of course you find it in essential oil. The ability of chamomile to relieve stress is also fairly well known, but it is only when the essential oil of Chamomile is distributed through a diffuser that you really begin to see some impressive results of chamomile aromatherapy.

As soon as you begin your diffuser routine you will find yourself becoming much calmer, in a short amount of time. For best results, just put 3 to 5 drops of chamomile essential oil into your diffuser and you will not have to worry about fatigue, anxiety, or depression during the winter months.

Lavender Oil

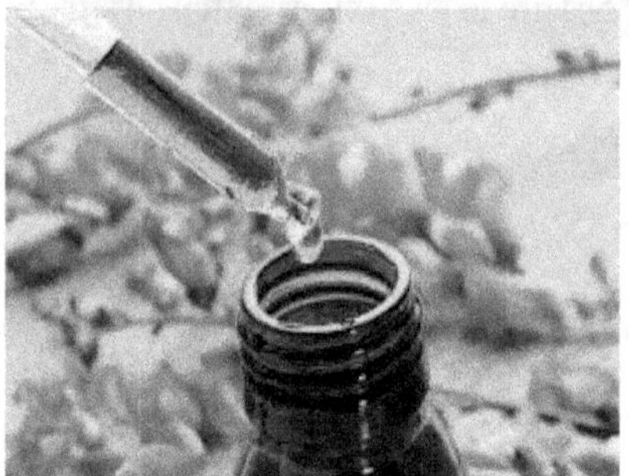

If you are feeling sluggish in the middle of January, this oil can get the blood pumping once again. When put in a proper diffuser, lavender oil reinvigorate the circulatory system, allowing for more oxygenated blood to flow to the brain. Bringing back much needed clarity and mental focus. Repeated exposure to the aroma of lavender wafting out of your diffuser over the course of the winter will help to safeguard you from those winter blahs.

Chapter 2: Essential Oils that Boost Metabolism and Weight Loss

Every single New Years, millions of people around the globe make their New Year's resolution to lose weight, and yet millions still keep the same weight, if not gaining even more by the end of the year! All of these people had good intentions; they just needed a little bit of a push in order to get them in the right direction. That push can come in the form of many essential oils that you can experience this spring to help you meet those weight loss resolutions once and for all!

Fennel Oil

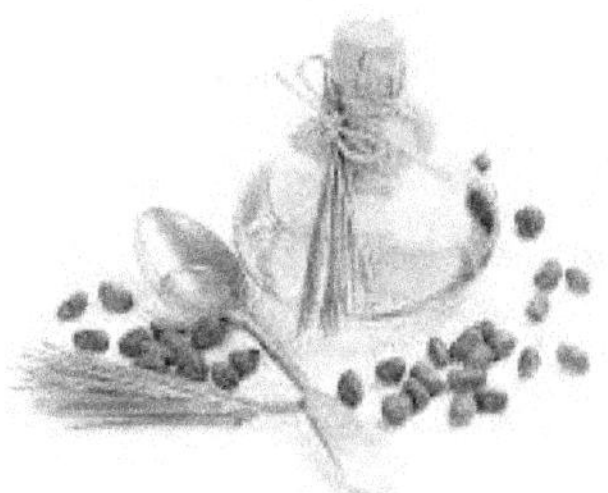

Placed in a diffuser, this essential oil has a very pleasant licorice smell. Breathing in this odor emanating from your diffuser, will instantly open up your lungs and allow you to breathe deeper, more oxygenated breaths. This more oxygenated lungful of air alone are enough to trigger your whole metabolic system into action.

After regular treatments your metabolism will be greatly sped up and weight loss can be much more easily achieved. I've known a lot of people that have used fennel as an additional supplement to their diet plan, and most have had wonderful results. In order to see immediate results, put 5 to 8 drops of this essential oil in your diffuser at least once a day.

Hawthorn Oil

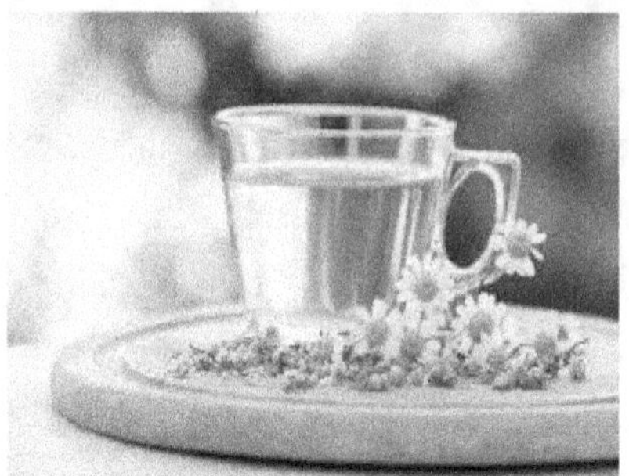

Hawthorne is a great essential oil to have on hand when the winter begins to turn to spring, due to its ability to completely invigorate your metabolism. As soon as you breathe in this essential oil as it gets pumped out of your diffuser, it quite literally goes straight to your heart. You see, hawthorn oil increases blood flow and greatly bolsters your heart's health. If you are having some issues with your heart you should give hawthorn a try. Because when you place a few strategic drops of this essential oil in your diffuser every day you will reap some great benefits.

Peppermint Oil

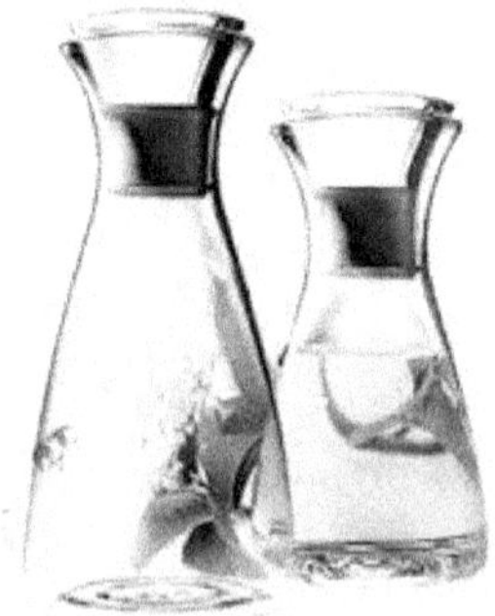

People are always surprised to hear that peppermint can boost the metabolism, but it's really no secret. After all, just take a look at all of those skinny, candy cane sucking elves at the North Pole! Now those guys are skinny! But in all seriousness, a few drops of peppermint oil evenly distributed through your diffuser can give your metabolism a very real and very significant boost.

You don't have to starve yourself to lose weight when your metabolism is revved up like this! After routine exposure to this essential oil, you should be able to greatly speed up the process of burning calories. Peppermint also helps to clear up any digestion issues, such as stomach bloat, or indigestion. So take this essential oil this winter in order to speed up your metabolism and you will lose weight.

Gurmar Oil

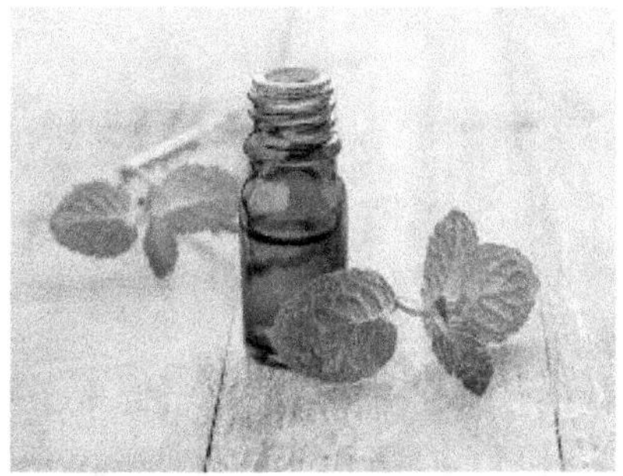

This essential oil is probably one of the least mentioned, and yet most underrated essential oils of all time. This essential oil has something called "gymnemic acid" inside of it that works hard to control your appetite and significantly boosts your metabolism. The whole metabolic process is sped up shortly after inhaling gurmar essential oil.

This is a great aid in losing weight anytime of the year, but the most famous aspect attributed to gurmar is its amazing ability to neutralize sugar cravings. So if you are having a hard time putting down all that candy from your Christmas stocking this winter, you might want to take a few good sniffs of gurmar essential oil in order to get rid of those cravings! This winter do yourself a favor! Sniff gurmar and lose weight!

Seaweed Oil

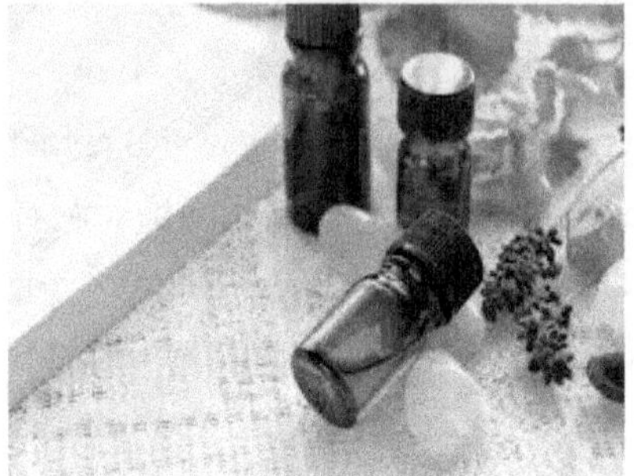

Seaweed oil has a phenomenal ability when it comes to speeding up your metabolism. It is due to the heavy iodine content in this oil working directly on your thyroid, that metabolism receives such a significant boost from this oil's dispersal.

There is an immediate metabolic reaction as soon as this aroma is inhaled. So if you are having any trouble at all keeping up with your commitments to lose weight this spring, you should definitely give this seaweed oil a try. It doesn't take much, just 2 or 3 drops of essential oil in your diffuser each day.

Grapefruit Oil

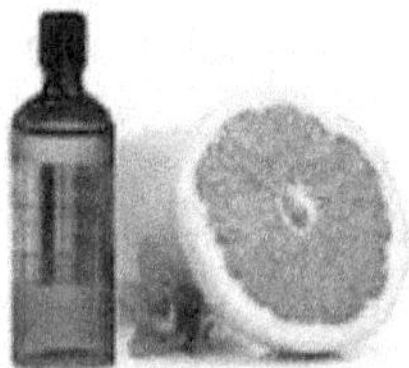

This oil comes from a rather tasty fruit, but grapefruit essential oil does much more than make for a tasty treat. This essential oil can actually speed up your metabolism and make you lose weight! This essential oil extracted from grapefruit when placed in a proper diffuser can have an immediate impact on the breakdown of fat in the liver.

When routinely breathed in, this oil eventually works to streamline your blood sugar levels while boosting your over all metabolism. Many diabetic patients have seen significant improvement after using this treatment. This spring, if you are trying to lose weight, this essential oil is a must!

Prickly Pear Oil

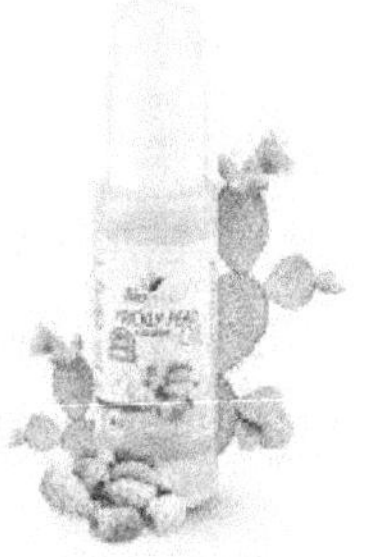

Hailing from the cactus family, this essential oil is extracted direct from the plant, with the oil pulled right from the pulp. Once extracted this essential oil is particularly potent, and when spread around the room by your diffuser on a regular basis, consider your metabolism as good as boosted! The effect of this boost is long lasting too, it doesn't just spike and then subside, it kicks it into high gear for the long haul. This extra metabolic boost will serve as a great help, as you make the transition from winter to spring.

Rosemary Oil

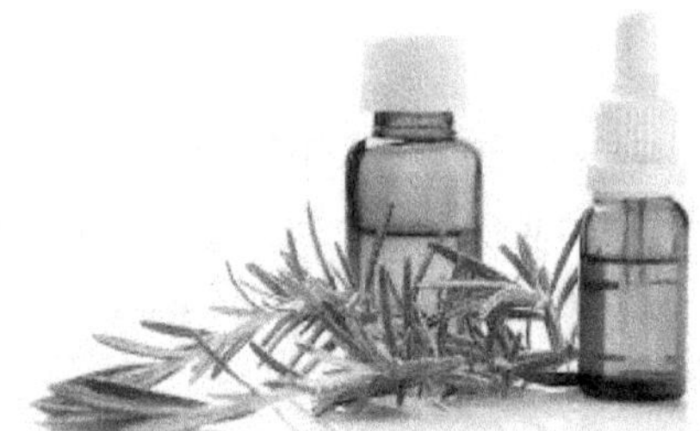

When this essential oil is inhaled through a diffuser it works on the body as a stimulant, immediately raising metabolism and aiding in that springtime weight loss. Thanks to rosemary essential oil you just might be able t fit in those skinny jeans again!

Besides being an aid to weight loss, rosemary has many other benefits such as strengthening the immune system and improving cognitive function. Rosemary is a natural muscle reliever as well, so while your metabolism is being boosted you can also ease those aches and pains! So go ahead! Give it a shot! Put rosemary oil in your own diffuser today!

Chapter 3: Wintertime Essential Oil for Your Immune System

Our Immune System is being constantly bombarded with outside threats and contaminants, and in the wintertime when the cold and flu season ramp up, it is absolutely under siege. Having that said, we should all do as much as we can to strengthen our natural immunity. And it just so happens that the use of essential oils is the best way that we can do just that.

Echinacea Oil

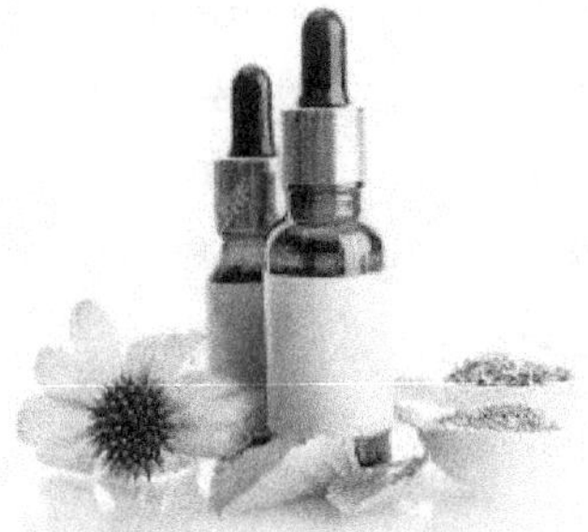

This essential oil has some amazing antibiotic and antiviral properties. All of this is great news for those of us trying to boost our immune system against the rigors of the cold and flu season during the months of winter. Echinacea has been used for thousands of years as a natural aid to the immune system. Native Americans used this very essential oil for hundreds of years to ward off sickness during the winter months. In order to boost your own immunity this winter, you should regularly use Echinacea essential oil as well. Typically 2 to 3 drops in the diffuser should suffice. Just make sure that your diffuser is operating in a place where you frequently breathe the air.

Astragalus Oil

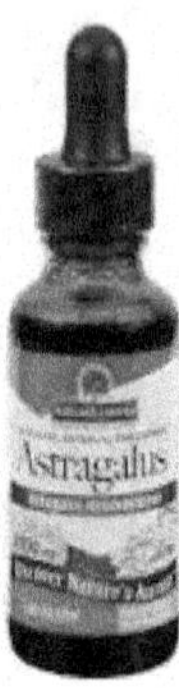

For many the winter is a time that really wears down on their normal immunity to illness. Astragulus oil however has stood the test of time as a natural immune booster. This oil has been around for thousands of years. It was used in China as a natural means of shielding the immune system from illness, and it could still be used for the same exact thing today. The immune system and astragalus are best friends, so you better not pass this opportunity of immune health up. Just put a few drops of this essential oil in your diffuser and you will be doing your immune system a big favor this winter!

Saffron Oil

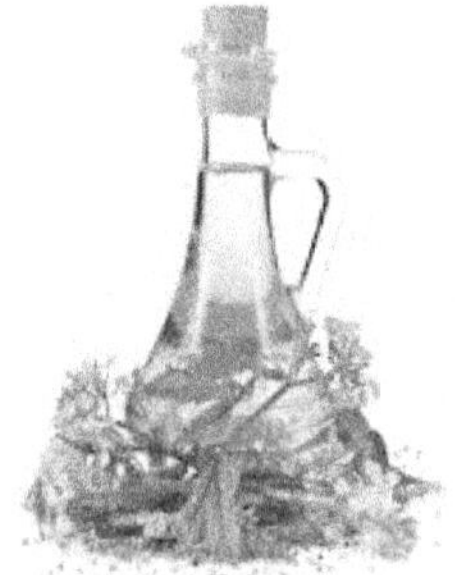

If you feel like your immune system is getting pummeled during the winter months, you might want to give saffron essential oil a try. This potent oil is extracted right out of the plant's stems with powerful immune boosting agents at its disposal. As soon as you breathe in saffron, the immune system is completely invigorated. Just drop this oil in your diffuser and you will start to feel a whole lot better in no time!

Oregano Oil

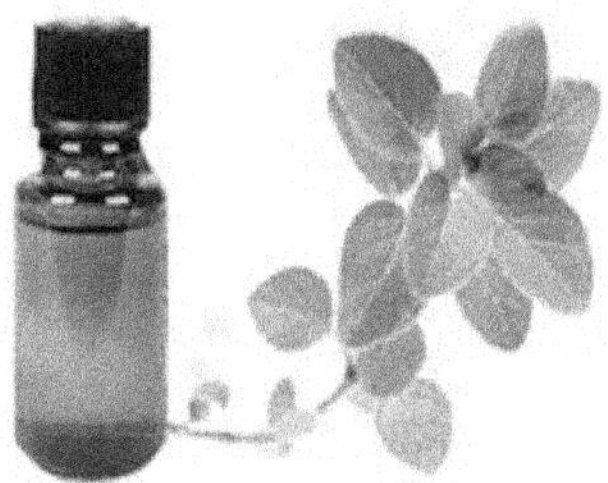

You may be more familiar with putting some oregano on your salad than with putting oregano in your diffuser, but this is an immune boosting essential oil that should not be missed! Oregano is absolutely loaded with antioxidants; these antioxidants can then take the roaming free radicals in our immune system to task, keeping our cells from being damaged, and providing more robust oxygen to our system. This serves to greatly boost our immune system, not allowing dangerous viruses, bacteria, and other harmful contaminants into our system.

Ginger Oil

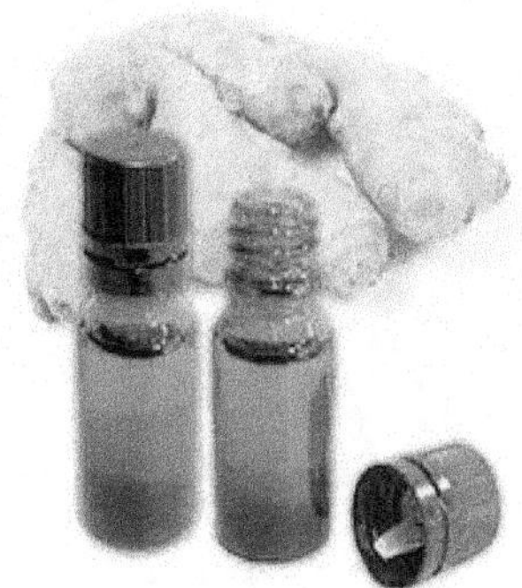

You might think of ginger this winter more in the context of gingerbread men, but this essential oil is also quite good at boosting your immune system. Ginger has natural anti-inflammation properties which work to strengthen general immune function. Outside contagion has a much harder time gaining access after you've been treated with ginger. Ginger also relieves aching joint pain, yet another great reason to give this essential oil a try!

Eucalyptus Oil

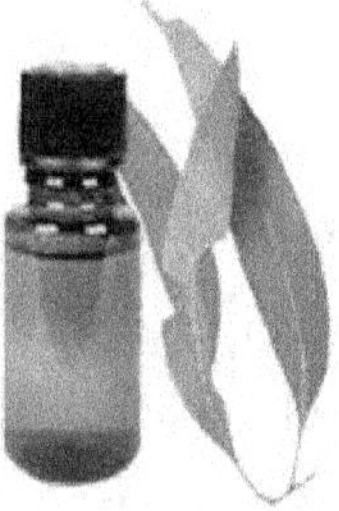

Be sure to put some Eucalyptus oil in your diffuser this winter, because this stuff immediately bolsters our immune system, as soon as we breathe it in. The aroma is pleasant, and it doesn't take much of it to make a difference in your immune health. So there is really no excuse not to give eucalyptus oil a try. Just add 1 or 2 drops of this essential oil to your diffuser and you will see a major difference in your immune health.

Chapter 4: Essential Oils for Heath All Year Round

There are so many uses for essential oils. So many in fact, that it is incredibly hard to list them all in one book! But I've compiled my best rudimentary list right here at the end of this book. In this chapter let's explore various essential oils that can be used all year round for a wide variety of purposes!

Cedar Oil

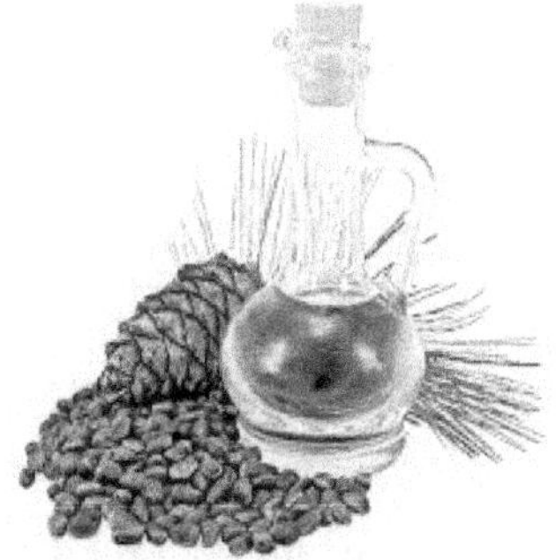

This essential oil blend is taking directly from the Cedrus Atlantica Tree and is well known for its use as a kind of hair tonic to ward off dandruff. In some instances, when applied to the scalp, it has even been known to be a good treatment for male pattern baldness. But when you place this essential oil in your diffuser it can do much more than bring you fuller, thicker hair.

This oil is known as a great cleansing agent, and can help tremendously with digestive issues. It's not real pleasant to talk about, but this essential oil is great at treating constipation. So if you are in need of some relief to your stomach issues, you might want to give cedar essential oil a try. This essential oil also seems to greatly improve the concentration and cognitive function of those who use it, so get your diffuser ready, and feel free to start a regular cedar oil routine.

Clary Sage Oil

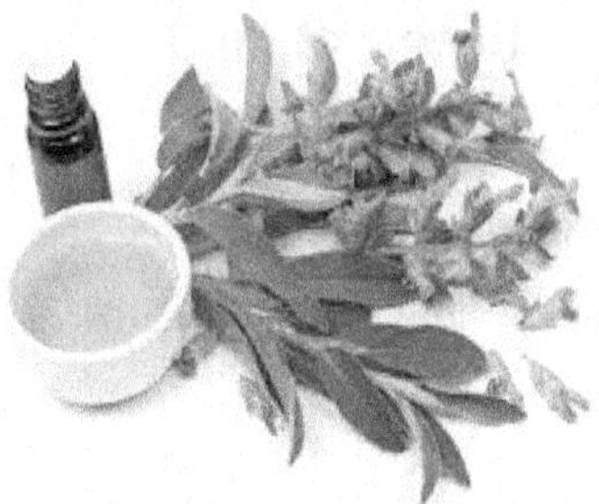

This oil tends to be expensive when you buy it from the health food store, but it is well worth it. Clary sage actually hails from France, but has been relocate to many other places across the globe. After putting this essential oil in your diffuser you will notice improvement in a wide variety of bodily functions such as better vision, digestion, as well as neurologic ability.

This should come as no surprise, since the name "clary" itself comes from the Latin word "clarus"; translated as literally, "clear eyes". This essential oil works wonders for tired and strained eyes. After long nights of typing and writing up my latest projects, I often resort to a little clary sage essential oil myself. Add this essential oil to your diffuser as soon as you can.

Thyme Oil

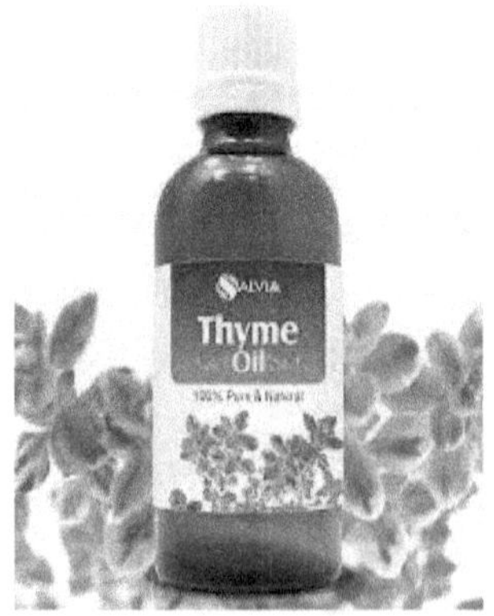

Thyme essential oil works as a natural antibacterial agent, as well as being an antispasmodic. Thyme naturally relieves the muscle tissue of the body and this includes the muscle tissue of the lungs when this essential oil is breathed into them. If you are having a particularly hard time breathing you should put a few drops of this powerful essential oil right into your diffuser and allow it to heal your breathing.

Lemon Oil

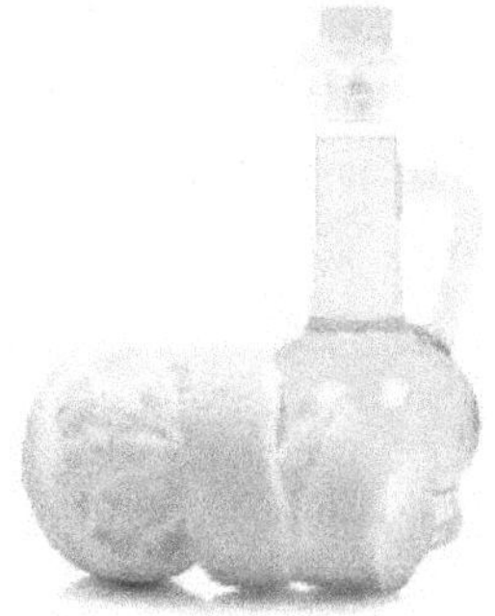

Lemon essential oil, just like cedar oil has been used quite extensively in hair products, in shampoos and lighteners, as a mean of enriching hair. It has several other uses however when you distribute this essential oil to a distributor. First of all, it is great at opening up the breathing passages, and when the aroma of lemon oil has been distributed across a wide area, it begins to work even faster. But along with your lungs, the carminative aspect of lemon essential oil greatly aids in digestion.

Patchouli Oil

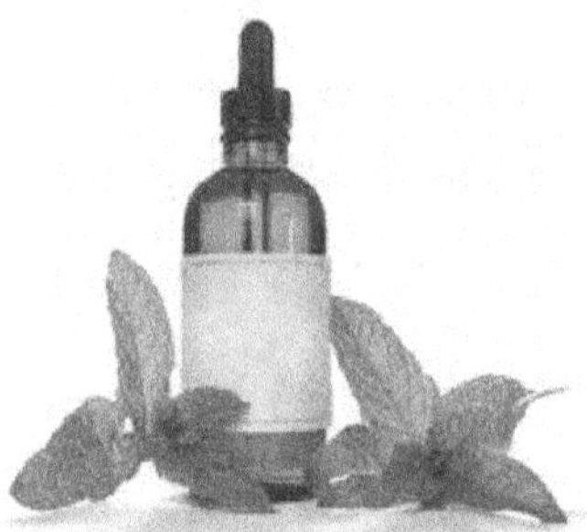

This one certainly harkens back memories of high school. I remember my senior year it seemed like my whole close had lathered up on this oil as a trendy kind of cologne. But much more than being just mere cologne, purely extracted Patchouli Oil when placed in your diffuser can do much to alleviate depression and anxiety. This is a benefit that you could certainly use all year round.

Vetiver Oil

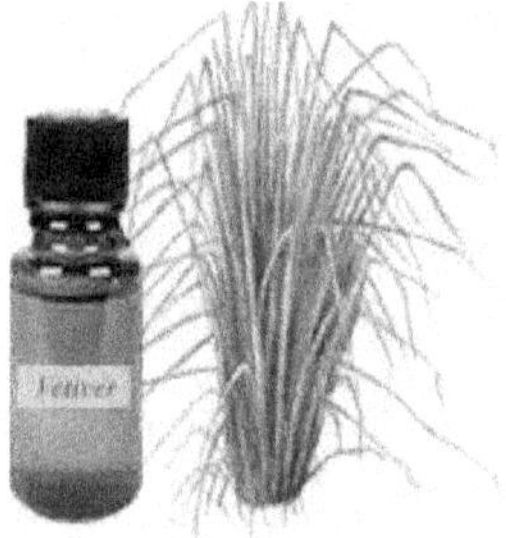

Vetiver works as an extremely powerful antiseptic but when it is placed in a diffuser it has several amazing cognitive uses as well. Because routine inhalation of vetiver essential oil can eliminate anxiety, get rid of mental fog, and greatly enhance over all mental cognition of those who expose themselves to its aroma. This essential oil is said to also enhance the immune system, so it is a welcome addition to anyone's oil diffuser routine.

Ylang Ylang Oil

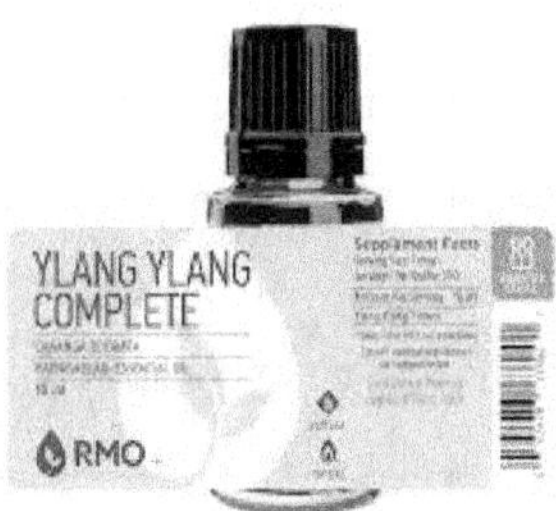

This essential oil is actually a great agent for restoring hormonal balance. Many women going through menopause use ylang ylang as a form of aromatherapy in order to get themselves into a more balanced state. This essential oil also works as a very efficient vasodilator widening the blood vessels and preventing those who use it from developing high blood pressure. Put about five drops of ylang ylang in your diffuser a day and you will be able to keep hypertension at bay!

Bergamot Oil

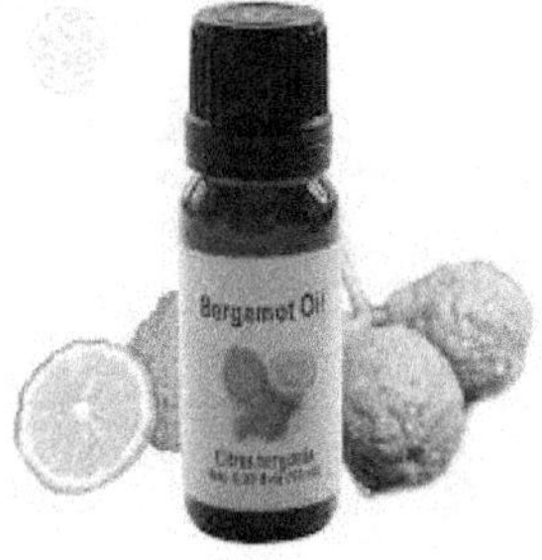

With a little bit of bergamot in your diffuser you can relieve much of your angst I a matter of seconds. The aroma is strong, and the nose is a powerful interface, so as soon as you breathe in the scent of this potent oil, it will go straight to your brain, slow down your racing heart, dry up sweaty palms, and alleviate your stress. Many have benefited from the powerful aroma of bergamot and in the aromatherapy circuit this essential oil is a number one draw.

In order to prepare your own exposure to this essential oil you should place 4 to 5 drops of bergamot oil in your diffuser and let the aroma gently waft up through your home. Besides helping you relax, this essential oil is good for other cognitive function as well. And if you are having trouble concentrating and you seem to be losing your memory and ability to recall, you may want to give bergamot essential oil a try.

This essential oil when inhaled through a diffuser on a daily basis has an amazing way of bringing back mental clarity and cognitive function. As the sweet smell of this oil is breathed in, so to is mental clarity, as anxiety and confusion are breathed out and eliminated! Try this essential oil any time of the year that you feel run down!

Coconut Oil

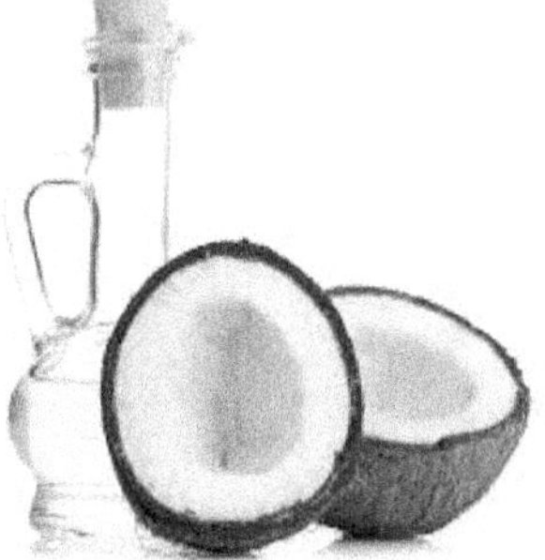

A regular diffuser routine of coconut oil is great for those that feel that their memory is starting to slip, because amazingly, studies have shown that a few drops of coconut oil dropped in a diffuser just might be able to get those synapses firing once again. In fact, coconut oil has been proven to be so successful that it has even been used to treat Alzheimer's disease. If you need a reset on your memory, don't hesitate to give coconut essential oil a try.

Basil Oil

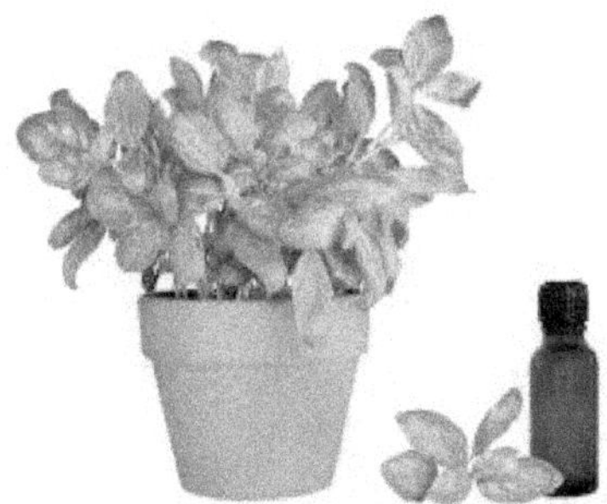

Basil oil seems to get the brain firing just fine after a few regular trips to the diffuser! The great thing about basil is that it seems to improve the retention of memory in those who inhale its aroma. I used to use basil essential oil myself back when I was in school. I used to breathe in its aroma right before I had big tests, and I always did seem to retain a lot more as result. So if your memory is bad, or your focus just needs a bit of sharpening you should seriously give this healing and restorative oil a try.

Cyprus Oil

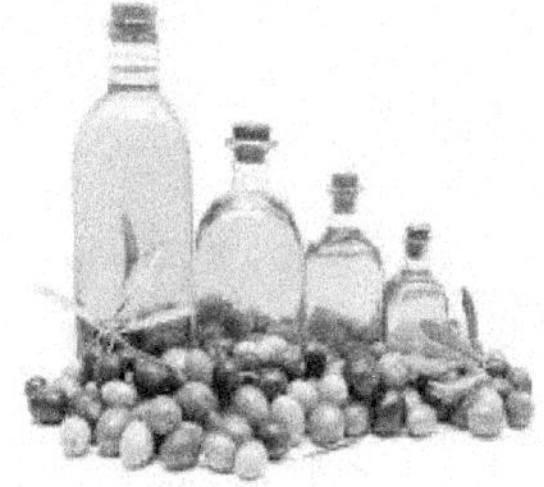

The smell alone is extremely refreshing, and as it turns out, the refreshing aroma of Cyprus oil can also refresh your memory. Cyprus has been proven to improve memory and other cognitive functions for those who routinely put this oil in their diffuser. Focus and mental clarity are greatly improved by this amazing essential oil. You can have a greatly expanded concentration all year round with cypress oil.

Coriander Oil

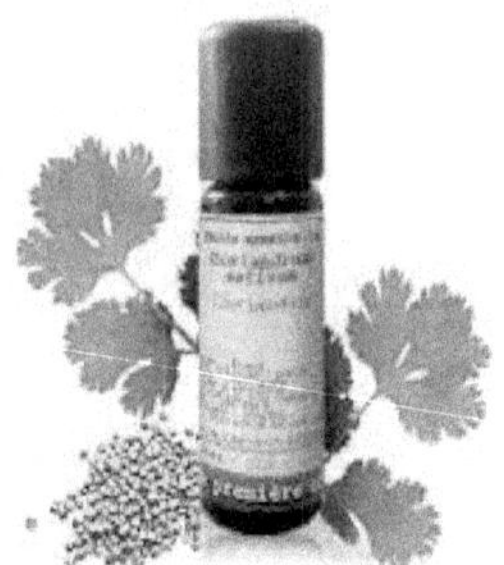

Coriander oil should really be called *cognitive essential oil* due to the amazing ability to restore memory, and improve concentration. When placed in a diffuser and used as routine aromatherapy, coriander oil directly stimulates the circulation of blood to the brain bringing important cognitive function right to the surface. With such a depth and reach like this, coriander oil should be used al year long.

Pine Oil

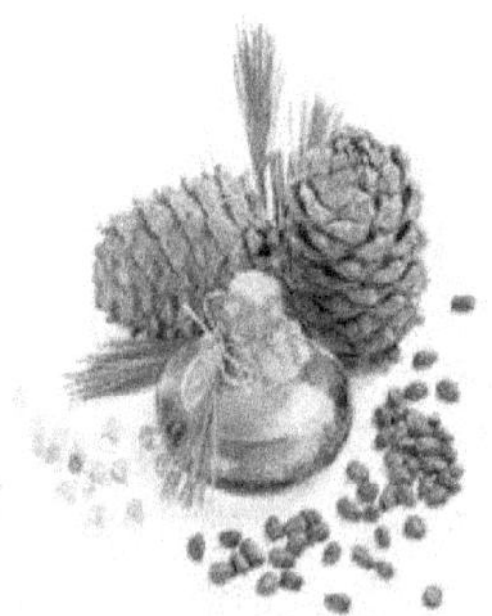

The aroma of pine when breathed through your diffuser on a daily basis can work as a muscle relaxer, easing muscle pain. It also tends to give those who are exposed to it a boost to their mental clarity. Helping to get rid of anxiety and fatigue, regular use of pine oil will give you just the boost of energy you need.

Sandal Wood Oil

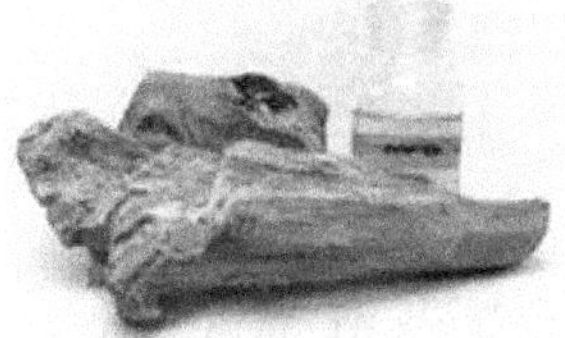

This essential oil has an amazing scent and when placed in a diffuser it can also have an amazing impact on your health. Hailing from ancient India this essential oil can freeze mental fatigue in its tracks, clearing the mind of anxiety, and giving you a brand new burst of energy to start your day. And in fact, that is exactly what you should do! In the morning liberally sprinkle 8 drops of sandal wood essential oil into your diffuser and breathe it in while you take your shower and get ready for your day. The aroma will perk you right up! It's even better than coffee!

Conclusion: Like A Well Oiled Machine

Most of us take good care of our cars, we change the spark plugs, add oil when we need to, and put gas in the fuel tank so we can get to our destination without a problem. But what about our very own physical body's? Who is going to take care of that? For many of us, our own physical heath goes by the wayside. But what if we could give ourselves a tune up?

What if all it took to jumpstart our system was the simple aroma of an essential oil coming through a diffuser? Well, as you have already ascertained from this book, that is exactly what we are driving at. It is through the use of essential oils that you can make sure your own body is in tip top shape and running smoothly like a well oiled machine.

FREE Bonus Reminder

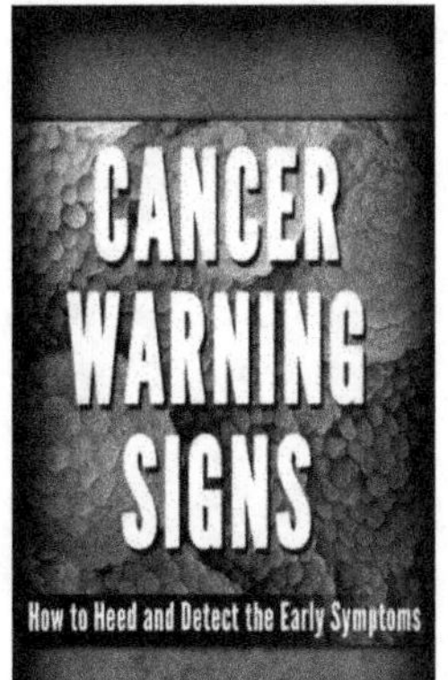

If you have not grabbed it yet, please go ahead and download your special bonus report *"Cancer Warning Signs. How To Heed & Detect The Early Symptoms!"*
Simply Click the Button Below

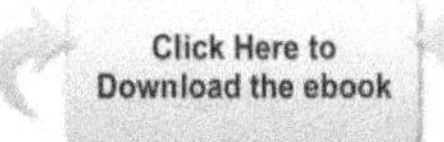

OR **Go to This Page**
http://healthylivingpeople.com/free/

BONUS #2: More Free & Discounted Books or Products
Do you want to receive more Free/Discounted Books or Products?
We have a mailing list where we send out our new Books or Products when they go free or with a discount on Amazon. Click on the link below to sign up for Free & Discount Book & Product Promotions.
=> Sign Up for Free & Discount Book & Product Promotions <=

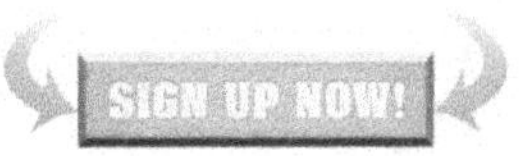

OR Go to this URL
http://zbit.ly/1WBb1Ek